Not Another Diet!
Losing Weight Without Exercise

By Shannon Challender

ACKNOWLEDGEMENTS

I would like to thank my family for their assistance with this book. They have collaborated with me to make this a better book. To them I say, "You guys are awesome".

TABLE OF CONTENTS

CHAPTERS

FORE WORD

While you read this book I would like you to remember, that I am not a medical professional. I write this book from the point of view of a lifelong dieter. I have spent my whole life working on one diet after another.

I have exercised on machines such as the stair climber, universal gym, rowing machine, and of course the dreaded treadmill at the local health club. I have put laps on the track and in the pool. I have played basketball and volleyball while at the recreation center on base. I've bought a number of home exercise equipment pieces. Such as the exer-cycle and the bow resistance flex machine. They have only ended up in storage collecting dust. Eventually I would get tired of moving them around and would try to sell them in a yard sale or put them on the classifieds section of the local paper.

I have tried exercise videos, books, and television exercise shows. Shows, where the exercise gurus spend hours working out on television where they attempt to sell you on their latest work out system. I have even purchased that ever so popular gaming system that comes with the whole kit and caboodle, including balancing pad and sport package. If you pay it the respect it requires, it will definitely make you believe you worked out.

Now, if this book was written by your local medical professional type, they would most likely be advising you to eat a balanced diet. I too would recommend a balanced diet. However, unlike the health professionals, I know that eating a balanced diet it is not always possible. For those persons that are not in the so called "middle class", feeding your family with fresh fruits and vegetables, is at times, next to impossible. The medical professionals want you to consume those healthy vegetables, fruits, proteins, and grains. Then they will tell you that you need a healthy dose of exercise. This book is not going to remind you to get plenty of exercise. The medical professionals do enough of that already. What you will find in this book is my opinion and my life of experience. After reading my opinion and description of my life stories, I hope you will gain some insight and a chuckle every now and again. If you want medical advice, please see your primary care physician.

Chapter One: Me

Welcome to my weight loss plan. First of all, I believe that there are those of you that have purchased this book in an effort to help you lose weight without exercising. Now it wouldn't be much of a book if I told you my secret at the beginning of the book. So I feel it is important to tell you a little about myself and what my life was like before I began to write this book.

As a way of introduction, I am a fifty four year old disabled Navy combat veteran. I spent my time in the Persian Gulf before the attack on September, eleventh, two thousand one. But I didn't write this book to boast about my military life and experiences, although, that might be a good read too.

I did most of my growing up in small towns all over the great state of Oregon. I was born the second oldest of four kids. I was the fair skinned, red headed, short little kid that had no discernable waist. This was a problem at times as I had nothing to keep my britches up. The whole time I was growing up, my family and I moved around a lot. It seemed that we moved every time my mother or step-father changed jobs, which was quite often. We moved so often that I attended thirteen schools in eight years. Because we moved so much, I never really had an opportunity to make friends. No sooner did we start school and begin getting to know our classmates, when it was time to move again. I couldn't really make friends, as I was rather shy. It takes a while to break into that shell of shyness that the timid children have. So for me, it was even harder since we moved around a lot.

So my best friend growing up was my little sister. There were sixteen months separating us. My oldest sister wanted to be in charge, so my little sister and I teamed up against her. I was short for my age, so my little sister and I were believed by most people to be twins. My mother took advantage of that and would buy us matching outfits. I remember one little set of cowboy pajamas. My little sister and I were ok with everyone thinking we were twins. Why shucks, she was kind of a tom boy anyway. I recall a time when we played outside with my trucks and cars in our city drawn in the dirt beneath the juniper trees of central Oregon.

Anyway, my mother and father divorced before I started creating memories. So growing up I didn't have a male father figure around to teach me how to play sports or how to fish or go hunting. Being shy, I didn't have any guy friends either. I didn't go out and play baseball, football, catch, or other outdoor sports most guys do with their fathers. Of course my mother would teach my sisters how to be young ladies, and just so I wouldn't be left out, I joined in with the girls. I learned to sew, knit, and crochet.

I also learned to listen. When my sisters or girl cousins played house or dress up with their dolls, I listened to the adults holding conversations. Most of the time they spoke of things that kids weren't meant to hear or be included in. The adults of my generation were of the old time belief that children should be seen and not heard. So I sat quietly and listened to their stories and did not exercise. Listening to their stories meant I sat around and just packed on the pounds. I believe it happens a lot to overweight kids.

These days' kids sit with the portable phone either glued to their ears or held 3 inches away from their faces texting. Then there are those that cannot stop staring at the monitor while playing the latest and greatest video game. They'll tell you it's because the super hero has just defeated the evil monster in level 12 and if they quit now they'll have to start all over. The point being if a person spends too much time sedentary, the pounds are bound to collect on the hips thighs and other places a person doesn't want it to show.

When I was about 6 years old, my mother remarried. He was a big burly guy that had been married before. He didn't necessarily like kids, save his own from his previous marriage. He treated my sisters and me very poorly. He liked to treat me as a proverbial red-headed stepchild. Matter of fact, I think that phrase was coined with me in mind. My step-father was an ex-con, and as such could only land migrant worker type jobs, such as fruit and vegetable pickers or logging. Turned out he was a great logger, but he was not such a great father figure. One day at the age of 13 my mother came to me and asked me if I would like to go stay with my biological father. Just until she could figure out what she was going to do about my step-father. She told me that she was either going to divorce him "or I don't know what". I left Oregon for California, and a week later, my mother called me in California and told me that my step-father had lost his life in a logging accident. He might have been a great logger, but apparently he didn't have much luck. It was like my mother had a premonition and she didn't want me to be exposed to him any longer. As I said, I attended thirteen schools before I decided to drop out of school and join the military.

Eventually I signed up with the United States Navy. They were always accepting recruits like me on the condition that I have a high school diploma or pass the GED exam. Because I sat and listened to the adults, I had more knowledge than your average seventeen year old. I was unemployed and had no other job opportunities or prospects at the time. The recruiter even offered to take me to the test. I passed the test, signed some papers and before I knew it I was on my way to boot camp in San Diego, California. Shortly after being assigned to a company as a seaman recruit, we started our physical fitness regimen. I got into trouble right off the bat. I was more than a match for the sit-ups and push-ups. However, the lack of outdoor activity showed in my performance during the endurance portion of the training.

I failed miserably at the two and a quarter mile run. It was required of all recruits to be completed in eighteen minutes or less. My time was nearer the twenty minute mark. Because of this, I was referred to the Fitness and Training squad (commonly referred to as the FAT squad by the other recruits of boot camp) where I was to remain until I was able to complete the run in under the required maximum time. I passed eventually and finally graduated boot camp. I had chosen my job in the Navy at the recruiters' office. The recruiter would ask you what you wanted to do and then give you something completely different. I wanted to be a dispersing clerk, a person that handles pay and other paperwork indoors. So my recruiter made me an Aircraft Maintenance Administrationman (AZ). A long title for a job that handles paperwork on changes and inspections on aircraft. After a short eight weeks in A school in Meridian, Mississippi, I received my first assignment to the fleet. My first squadron was Antarctic Development Squadron Six (VXE-6), home ported in Point Mugu, California.

The roll of VXE-6 was that of support for the National Science Foundation. Our squadron was assigned to basically be the local delivery trucks of the southern most hemisphere. In that roll VXE-6 made six month deployments to New Zealand and McMurdo Station, Antarctica. The reason for our being in Christchurch, New Zealand, was so we could take care of the regular maintenance and inspections required by the navy. Particularly those maintenance and inspections that could not be done in the severe cold of Antarctica. When those inspections were complete and any necessary repairs or maintenance was also complete, the aircraft would be loaded with supplies and flown to McMurdo Station Antarctica.

Once I settled down to my new job in the squadron, I started making friends of my fellow shipmates. Some of my shipmates wanted to be as helpful as possible. They were ever so happy to fill me in on what would happen to me upon my first deployment to McMurdo, and it wasn't something the welcome wagon would do. Upon my first trip to the southern station of McMurdo, I would get to experience the initiation into the "Old Antarctic Explorer" brotherhood. I would become an OAE. Such considerate shipmates told me stories of what they had endured during that initiation, most of it I believe was embellished, which scared this seventeen year old sailor nearly to death. There was of course, a way to avoid this scary initiation I was told. All I would need to do was gain enough weight and the Navy would kick me out. This way I wouldn't have to worry about the initiation. Well, after hearing that, I figured I could gain enough weight and the Navy would be happy to rid themselves of me. Besides I didn't have any problem gaining weight. Hey, to a young sailor this sounded like the easy way to avoid the perils of initiation. As a young man, I did not know that one day I would love the Navy and my time in service to my country. Regardless of that, I spent the next four months eating every doughnut, candy bar and cheese burger I could get my hands on.

In that four months I was able to go from a reasonable one hundred sixty four pounds to a miserable one hundred ninety two. (A weight I would love to be at today.) Much to my dismay, this did not get me out of this much dreaded deployment. It did however get me assigned to the squadron mandatory fitness program. Now I was really in hot water. Not only was I overweight, but I was still going on deployment and I had to face that dreaded initiation.

The rest of my Navy career was spent dieting, exercising, making weigh-ins, and worrying about when they would expel me. I found that gaining the weight was the easy part. Getting the weight off was a lot harder than I had anticipated. But I wasn't thinking about that when I enjoyed those oh so many doughnuts, candy bars, and cheeseburgers.

About a year after my first enlistment was up. I met and married a woman that was the Mississippi State Queen for the "Take Off Pounds Sensibly" (TOPS) weight loss group. She had lost one hundred four pounds that year to reach her goal weight. At six foot one and a hundred eighty four pounds, she was a striking woman. After two years of marriage our daughter was born. My wife and I spent the next eighteen years fighting weight issues. We tried all manner of diets and exercise routines, to no avail.

During this time I discovered the will power to quit smoking. I used a system of will power and replacement therapy. I changed all the habits I had that included smoking. For instance, whenever I got in my vehicle, I would light a cigarette. So, the first thing I changed was vehicles. I started replacing the cigarettes with breath mints. I figured I could break the habit of smoking and get an additional benefit of fresher breath. It seemed to work well and within a month I had ceased smoking. Will power got me through some hard times. Well, will power and an empty wallet that is. It's amazing what you can do when your pocket book is empty.

After some difficult times with my wife of twenty years, she and I agreed came to an agreement that we should divorce. A year of being single and I found a wonderful woman in the great state of Texas. She believes me to be her knight in shining armor. I thought that she was the one that should be placed on a pedestal. She was the preacher's daughter, babysitter, lifeguard, part-time teacher, short order cook, and mother of two boys. She is a beautiful woman, a little overweight, and she had a truck. In the Great State of Texas it's almost as important to have a truck as it is to learn the language. You have to learn TexMex and drive a truck or you just aren't a "proper" Texan.

During the next eight years the two of us fought our weight problems together without much success. The older I became, the more weight I put on. But try as I might the weight went on but did not come off. With medical problems mounting and with every year I aged, my increasing weight just made things worse. That's when I had an epiphany.

Chapter Two: Dieting

So now that you know a little about me, you may be able to understand where I get the chutzpah to write this book about dieting. I am not a dietician, nor am I a medical professional. However, I have spent thirty something years dieting, counting calories, carbohydrates, and pounds. I have been watching my weight so long, I could probably get a degree in nutrition just by testing out. I have learned a lot about foods, calories, and dieting from all the dieticians and doctors I have had the pleasure to meet over the years. If you want a list of foods, and amounts of foods, you will need to seek out a dietician. This is my story, and again, I am not certified or licensed to provide any professional help.

I have had a real hard time with skinny people telling us vertically challenged people, what to eat and how much you can have. Sure skinny people can tell you what you should eat, but if you have ever eaten the foods they want you to eat, you will eat things that you probably don't like. Let's face it, most of the skinny people have high metabolisms and don't need to read a book like this. Even the First Lady has gotten in on the "eat good food" band wagon. The newest thing is changing the food pyramid into a plate. I haven't read any of this new propaganda about the amounts they want you to eat. But you can be assured that it will include the four basic food groups.

What is on the diet you ask? Veggies. Green, yellow, and red ones such as asparagus, carrots, celery, tomatoes, peas, tofu, bean sprouts, cauliflower, spinach, blah, blah, blah. Most of these foods are missing the one essential item that gives most foods flavor. Fat. Most foods taste good because of the fats they contain. In the meat or protein group there is fish, chicken, tofu, portabella and other types of mushrooms, calamari, oysters, peanut butter, etc. In the grain group, we have 7 grain bread, made of what I call nuts and twigs, all of which come in usually very small portions of whatever the grain de jour is for that moment. But for goodness sake, you had better not include any glutens, which is found in almost everything.

Then there is the diary group. I call this the yummy group because it includes cheese, butter, cream, etc. But the food police don't want you to eat these foods because there is so much fat, besides the nutritionist would rather you eat the veggies and nuts and twigs. It seems to me that only a goat, a cow, or other grass eating animals would want to eat the kind of food they recommend. I am sure you noticed the continued reference to tofu? I think the producers of tofu must sit on the board of all food group administrators. I find it hard to believe anyone in their right mind would want to eat tofu intentionally. It is said that tofu takes on the flavor of the foods it is combined with. I don't know about you, but I would like to disagree. Maybe it does, maybe it doesn't. I prefer to believe the latter.

Now, I am not a person that believes exercise does not have any place in the world of weight loss, but my disabilities tend to limit the types of exercises that I can do. So that is what made me try this life style change. So now, if you are ready for me to get to the diet part, here it is.

Chapter Three: Eating

My weight loss plan consists of primarily two things. First of all, reducing what you eat. By that I mean reducing the amount of what you eat. I believe most people have become over-weight due to the excess food they have consumed over a life of poor food choices. I know this is true of me. For years I have just eaten what I wanted when I wanted it. That type of diet does not work when you are on a fixed income. Of course there are those people that have glandular anomalies, which make it next to impossible to either gain weight or lose weight. Let's face it if you do not have any medical complications, you should be able to lose weight with this diet. Please make sure you consult your primary physician before starting any diet.

You most likely became over-weight by over indulgence of the foods a thin person would avoid. Am I right? That is how I got my excess weight. I did not exercise enough and I ate too much. When I wanted to lose weight, I just had to reduce the amount of food that passed between my teeth. I could not seem to stick to the traditional diet, as I love breads, beef, and pork and all that other creamy goodness that comes from milk and cheese.

However, I also learned some interesting things about my body when I started this particular diet plan. I found that if I stopped eating breads with yeast, I was not nearly as miserable. But I found I can consume breads that are not made with yeast. Such as the biscuits that come in a tube in your grocer's cooler, near the eggs. Another thing I found is that even though breads that are made with yeast but have been cooked thoroughly, such as pizza dough is ok. If I choose thin crust pizza, it is not as heavy and I believe the yeast is cooked out and won't bother my digestion.

I found that this was true about milk as well. I am of the belief that milk disguises itself as a liquid when in fact it is actually a solid or at least becomes solid when it mixes with the human body. I am no expert in chemistry or science. I am just giving you my layman's opinion. So even though I love milk, I have stopped consuming milk whenever I can. Of course a lot of food contain milk and I am not saying I will avoid milk like that, I just don't drink it. I'm not saying I'm lactose intolerant either. Just the opposite, I love milk. I think it is healthy for people to drink, with all the vitamins. Now I ain't sayin' it is and I ain't sayin' it ain't. But don't you get full very quickly when you drink milk? Therefore, milk must be a solid once it combines with stomach acid, right?

Second thing I have employed in my diet is will power. I found I had the will power to quit smoking some fifteen years ago, so I believed that I still had that ability. I would just need to rekindle that ability, and focus it on reducing my consumption of food and I could stop over-eating.

What do skinny people have that we over-weight people don't? The skinny people have either a high metabolism rate or they have and use the will power to keep from over eating. For instance, have you ever heard a skinny person say "No thanks, I'm not hungry", when you offer to buy them lunch? I deduced that since I do not have a high metabolism, I would have to rely on will power. This is the hardest thing I have ever done or had to do. If you are one of those people who like to exercise, by all means, do so. I would suggest you add exercise to any diet. Exercise can help weight fall off.

A few years ago, I took up bicycle riding. But because I was so large, I could not ride one of those regular bicycles. So, I chose a bicycle that resembled a recumbent exercise bike. I found the seat was much more comfortable than those saddles that look like a ping pong paddle. If you ever saw me riding a standard bicycle it would look like the saddle had gone some place where the sun doesn't shine. The bike I purchased had a shock absorber and made for a much smoother and generally a better ride. It's a little tricky to get used to riding, but once you have it mastered, the ride is very comfortable. I thought the ride was so nice I once rode a hundred miles in one day. Even though recumbent bicycles have lots of gears, they are not all that easy to ride up any hill. My bicycle had twenty four gears, and if you shifted to 1st gear, you might be pedaling like you were going crazy, and the bicycle would fall over, because you are not moving fast enough to stay upright (just kidding). Even going downhill they have some unstable characteristics. I found if I exceeded a certain speed downhill, the bicycle would start wobbling and give me the shakes. (Pun intended). But if you have a flat surface to ride on, it is very easy to ride. If you aren't into exercising, or just plain can't exercise, then you'll have to use pure will power to lose weight.

So think of will power as clothing. When you go into a clothing store and find a beautiful shirt and you absolutely won't wear that color, you use your will power to say "I am not wearing that". That is will power. It's the same thing with food. You'll have to use your will power in order to say no to the excess food. However, putting your will power in action to reduce your intake of food can actually be more difficult than convincing yourself to be physically active. I say this because exercising your will power to reduce your weight and not over-eat, is a sixteen-hour a day effort. I say sixteen hours, because I sleep about eight hours a day. If you don't rest you may not get the results you seek. So make sure to get your rest.

I believe in rest. You have to give your body some down time so you can recharge your energy levels. I personally try to get at least eight hours of rest and you don't have to think about food while you're sleeping. Besides, if you aren't allowing your body the rest it needs, you will have a harder time losing weight than those persons that do get the proper amount of rest. Now the proper amount of rest is an issue that is debated by experts. I believe that the proper amount of rest is the amount that your body requires. If you sleep long periods of time, you may have issues that need to be discussed with your physician. If you sleep very short periods of time, then you also may need to talk to your doctor. I usually sleep eight hours a day. If you need eight hours of sleep, and you need to get up at 7:30 am, you'll have to go to bed at 10:30 pm not midnight, like some kids now days do. Well anyway, if you get the proper amount of rest, your body will thank you. Which will make it easier to get that extra weight off.

My diet, which is not actually a diet, is more of a life style change. All I have done is just reduce what I eat. I think that most dieticians will tell you to limit certain foods in your efforts to lose weight. In this, I would agree. Although, I am not a dietician, there are times even I agree with them.

I say you don't have to eat special foods for breakfast, lunch and dinner, just pay attention to how much the food you do eat weighs and try to keep it to a minimum. The longer you keep this up, the better you will get at figuring out which food will work best for you and which foods you should stay away from.

This is where the will power comes in handy. The only difference between losing weight and gaining weight is, the amounts of food you eat at any given sitting. If you can channel your will power into the effort to reduce what you eat, you will be shedding pounds so quick you may need to buy new clothes every month. I am not a person that loves to buy clothes all the time, but when you can pull out one of those belts you haven't been able to wear for a while, and it fits again. That makes you want to go show someone. My wife and I have been working on this diet for a while and she loves to buy new clothes. Me, I would rather not have to go clothes shopping until they look like they are hanging off me.

Now to implement this diet plan, I started thinking of it this way. I would not cut out any food, except those that my body doesn't like. All my life I have been an advocate of listening to your body. Usually when you are out and about in the family vehicle, or just thinking of stopping for something to eat, listen to what your body is asking for. I believe that your body is very good at telling you what it wants or needs in order to correct some deficiency in your body. In this case your body might tell you it wants Italian or Greek or some Asian food. I would just gage what the food weighed and consume a portion that did not weigh very much. I would just use my built in judgment and eat smaller amounts of the heavy foods and a little more of the foods that are lighter. I am not telling you to eat three ounces of this or four ounces of that. What I am saying is you should use your own judgment. If you feel guilty about eating too much of it, then you probably should substitute something that weighs less. You will feel much better about this new life style change if **you** make the decisions about what food to consume and what food to eat less of. Only you can prevent forest fires. At least that is what Smokey the bear used to say. But if you employ this will power life style change, you are the only person responsible for your success or failure.

Now there are some foods I found that are good and some that are not so good. I live on a limited income. I cannot afford to go to the grocery store at a moment's notice and get fresh veggies, and I know that there are plenty of you that also cannot go shopping on a moment's notice. The boxed foods are those that when combined with hamburger or chicken make a meal. For my family, they are still nearly a daily meal for me and my family. These are the heavy foods though. I usually take smaller portions of these. However, we usually have a canned vegetable, such as green beans, or corn as a vegetable. That is where I would load my plate. If you have ever been to a dietician, you will remember they stress plenty of vegetables. The reason they stress vegetables is because they are so good for you and they have nearly zero calories, not to mention they are high in fiber. If in doubt though, go heavy on the veggies and stay away from the heavier foods loaded with carbohydrates.

If someone brings or makes desert, don't worry. Just remember that even in the desert world, heavier foods are the ones that are the worst for you calorie wise. Calories are something I don't worry about much. You'll go nuts trying to count all those calories. If I apply my heavy foods are bad theory, then you should be able to get rid of the calories. A real favorite around my house for desert, for example, is Angel Food Cake with fresh sliced strawberries. It makes you feel like you are getting something yummy. But it is lighter than other forms of sweet foods and the strawberries are good for you in the calorie department. The fruits are almost free foods no matter the weight.

One of the other foods that I feel are good, are the yogurt food group. I'm probably the only one that thinks of it that way, but hey, chocolate is also a food group. If you can stand to eat the reduced fat version of yogurt, do it. It is by far the best in the yogurt group.

Chapter Four: Water

I have saved this chapter for last. This chapter will be devoted to one of the most key things about this life style change. Water. It is something the body is made up of. It may be one of the heaviest things you can put in your mouth. Water weighs in at approximately eight pounds per gallon. But when it comes to losing weight, water is one of the most important things you can consume. Well, water and or liquids. Believe it or not, water was the subject of the PC police just the other day. I heard on the radio that there are advertising agencies that are giving water the big push. Companies are out there trying to make a lot more money off people becoming healthier, and charging more for it. Anyway, water will fill you up and it has less calories than any food mentioned in this book or any other.

Let me put this question to you. If your driveway became covered in dirt, how would you clean the mess up? Well, let me help. You might use a broom but that would take a long time. Most people would grab the garden hose, turn on the water and wash that dirt off their driveway. Would you throw a single bucket of water at it? No, of course you wouldn't. The same goes for food you eat. Once in your body, the food is like that. It's something messing up your driveway. The best way to wash it out of your body is consume lots of water. Once the water goes over your lips, it starts washing the junk out of your colon. But one glass of liquid just won't do it. You have to get mass quantities of water. However, don't try sticking a garden hose in your mouth, as this could cause any number of physical problems. But definitely continue drinking glasses of water or fluid of your choice all day long. Once your body is done removing the valuable components from the food, what is left is just waste. You need to get rid of that junk. Wash it out!

Now there are some people that believe that liquid HAS to be water and nothing else would do. However, I don't care to drink plain water. I like water to some degree. But I would prefer to add one of those little tea mixes such as tea/lemonade mix. You may like coffee or some sort of juice drink. I would suggest that if you want it to work best, the liquid you consume should be some sort of low sugar or sugar free drink. I suggest something as close to water as you can get.

I have seen people that have tried to drink only diet soda. I used to myself, but I was never able to get enough weight off or keep it off while I was drinking diet soda. Also, there is a lot of stuff in sodas that I wouldn't recommend you drink. Besides, water is cheaper most of the time. I once heard that a person needs to drink eight glasses of water a day plus an additional glass of water for each 10 pounds you have to lose, or some such thing. Personally I think a person should drink what a person can hold. Don't make yourself sick drinking.

I once heard of a person out in southern California that died of water poisoning. I didn't even know that was possible until I heard that story. Apparently this woman had entered one of those radio call in shows about "What would you do to get tickets to the local concert". Most things you overdo will come back to bite you.

But always remember, whatever you put in your driveway, has to be washed out with something. You shouldn't wash your drive way with something that can dirty it up even more than it was when you started.

EPILOGUE

There you have it. I have spilled the proverbial beans and told you the secret of my success. You can try it for yourself, but you have to be honest with yourself. If you cheat, you are the only one that will know. If you cheat you don't hurt anyone but yourself. You can't blame anyone else. I call this my lifestyle change. So maybe the secret in all this is don't try to diet. Change the things in your life that cause you to gain weight. This lifestyle change will take a while to remove your weight. You most likely didn't put the weight on overnight, so don't expect it to come off overnight.

Please remember, I hear it all the time. "Before you start any weight loss program you should consult your physician to ensure you are healthy enough to begin this life style program".

Here's wishing you the best in your quest for weight loss. Remember you can do it.

www.ingramcontent.com/pod-product-compliance
Lightning Source LLC
Chambersburg PA
CBHW070939290526
45795CB00003B/1073